Eating Disorders in Pregnancy

How to beat the odds and avoid relapse

By Barbara Kiersz Mueller, DO, IEC, CFMDL-1

*Dedicated to my children. You make me want to be
a better person every day, to set an example for you
and stay grounded and connected to my wise mind.
I hope to break the family patterns. You will still
have your own trials and tribulations in your life, a
lot of them because of me, but I hope none are due
to the things I've tried so hard to improve.*

Introduction

I considered myself fully recovered from my eating disorder for three years (quasi-recovered for another three years before that) before getting pregnant. My husband and I were fortunate to plan our pregnancy. I knew it would come with some self-image challenges, but I didn't anticipate relapsing after being free from the prison of my own mind for so long.

The prenatal paperwork at the obstetrician's office was pretty standard and, as I expected, it asked about any history of eating disorder. This is for multiple reasons, one of them being ruling out any current eating disorder that could potentially harm the baby due to maternal malnourishment. However, I learned that mentioning a past history of eating disorder didn't come with receiving any education of the statistics of eating disorder relapse in pregnancy. I learned this on my own after another friend with history of eating disorder who had been fully recovered for years also had lapses during her pregnancy:

67% of women with a history of eating disorder will relapse during pregnancy, and 50% will relapse during the postpartum period[1]. There isn't much research on this topic as it would be potentially unethical to have a woman maximize eating disorder thoughts during a pregnancy as it could risk the baby's life. So, it is natural that we don't have so much data on this topic. Additionally, a lot of us feel ashamed and guilty that we have these thoughts after years in recovery, and we may not be inclined to share it with our loved ones that we are having disorder thoughts again. Most of our loved ones will assume that we've surpassed our eating disorder and are done with it, just like that. But we know that it's a lifelong struggle, even fully recovered. The thoughts my lurk and show up when we least expect them. Pregnancy is no exception.

Recovering from an eating disorder is difficult and requires a multi-provider approach including therapists, doctors, and nutritionists, to provide the best chances of recovery. Recovery is so hard, only a third of people with an eating disorder recover (citation). Imagine your self-disappointment and shame when you relapse in pregnancy without any prior warning.

I wrote this book in hopes of normalizing relapse of eating disorders during pregnancy by sharing my own story and adding tips that helped me during my pregnancy in order to help achieve full recovery once again.

Weeks 1-6

You've missed your period.

If you planned this pregnancy, you're probably counting down the days until you can take a home pregnancy test and confirm your bundle of joy is on the way. Hormones are shifting and you may potentially develop constipation at this point, maybe some mild bloating, but typically not much else. Joy and eagerness consume your day.

You are finally able to pee on a stick and get your (+) or (||) confirming your pregnancy.

You set up your initial OB appointment for 8 weeks.

Most likely, you like planning, certainty, and having control of situations (after all, eating disorders thrive with these types of personalities). You are proud of yourself for being prepared and ready.

Anticipation starts building as you approach your OB appointment, and you are ready to officially confirm the pregnancy with an ultrasound. As soon as you get that second confirmation, you start planning your baby registry, the nursery, sleeping arrangements, and visualize holding your tiny miracle in your arms.

Weeks 6-12 (sometimes beyond)

Nausea kicks in.

Potentially, at this point, your eating disorder thoughts suddenly reappear from out of the blue. You were not expecting this. The bloating is getting worse, and you notice your body changing. You realize you have no control over your body for the next nine months (and no control over your son or daughter EVER). Be it a mix of hormones and a mix of the eating disorder thriving with lurking uncertainty, you find yourself ruminating about how grateful you are that you're nauseous so that you abstain from eating.

Or you may find yourself in a completely different situation. You are so nauseous, you can't even think about food, or your body, or work, or anything else for that matter. All you can think about is getting relief from the nausea.

Personally, nausea is my kryptonite. I am able to tolerate pain. I am resilient to get through recovery. But nausea... I can't handle it. I personally took **vitamin B6 25-50mg three times a day**[2] **and alternated between peppermint and ginger drops**. I dislike ginger, but I absolutely cannot stand nausea. So, I would push through the ginger taste just to get relief from the queasiness. **Another thing you can pair with vitamin B6 to help with nausea is doxylamine 10-12.5mg three times a day**[3].

My first pregnancy was a miscarriage, so I avoided taking anything that wasn't a vitamin. I found myself in scenario A. The level of anxiety and uncertainty about whether I could carry a pregnancy to term was all-time consuming. There was not a second in the day I wasn't thinking about this. My eating disorder saw this as an opportunity to start whispering in my brain, reappearing after years of being dormant. Initially, I didn't even realize it was ED in my brain. My anxiety was so bad, that having those thoughts about being glad I wasn't eating were barely even helping with the anxiety. Let alone me realizing what was actually starting to redevelop in my brain.

Weeks 12-20

The belly starts to grow.

By this time during my pregnancy, every day that went by in which I felt my uterus slightly larger, I would feel a second of relief from anxiety. Yes, I checked my fundus size (medical term for the top of your uterus) and measured how much closer it was to the bellybutton, which is typically achieved by week 20. This compulsion was very similar to body checking during my eating disorder. At the time, I did not make such connection (my therapist did immediately). But I did know it was a compulsion to help ease my anxiety about possible miscarriage again. I would have daily flashbacks of the day I passed our first fetus in the toilet after taking misoprostol. By this time of the second and third pregnancies, I had contacted a therapist who specialized in pregnancy losses who also had experience with eating disorders as I did start getting concerned about my body changing. Notice the paradox: I was yearning and praying for my uterus to keep growing as reassurance that the baby was doing well, and, at the same time, I was starting to get anxious about my body changing, most likely irreversibly.

Simultaneously, the nausea subsided around week 14 for me and I became ravenously hungry. The combination of nausea, body changes, and constant hunger, led to more eating disorder fears, and I started reverting to some disordered eating, trying to find some form of control in a completely uncontrollable situation. I **sought out professional help** immediately.

I knew how difficult it had been for me to recover from my eating disorder the first time around, and I was not about to have a baby and then have to go through recovery again. I didn't want to put myself through that as a new mom. But most of all, I wanted to **set an example for my unborn child**. I grew up with a mom with an eating disorder and I was (and am) adamant about breaking the generational eating disorder cycle. As soon as I started sensing my concerns about my changing body, I contacted the therapist to help me cope with the anxiety without falling back on my eating disorder behaviors.

If you notice yourself having even the slightest disordered eating or body dysmorphic thoughts, don't wait to contact a therapist. I personally contacted a therapist that had previously been in my treatment circle, and she suggested someone who also had experience with pregnancy loss. I contacted her and met with her weekly. It was not covered by insurance and sessions were expensive. But that didn't matter to me; I needed to get my ED thoughts under control for the same of my unborn baby. I wanted my baby to develop in a healthy womb environment: nourished and at peace.

My second pregnancy was different. This time around, I knew my body was capable of carrying a pregnancy through term. But the anxieties around the body did come up again. I thought that having gone through pregnancy body changes one time around would prevent the disordered thoughts the second time. But they showed up differently each pregnancy.

Independently and individually, we have as much risk of relapsing subsequent pregnancies as we do the first one. In fact, the disorder thoughts started showing up earlier for me during my second pregnancy, as my belly started growing earlier in the pregnancy. I started showing 10 weeks before my prior pregnancy. When I was four months pregnant in my second pregnancy, my belly looked as it did when I was six months with my previous pregnancy. ED decided to take this as an opportunity to start whispering in my head that I should do something about this. That I should make sure I didn't gain weight. That I could potentially develop metabolic conditions in pregnancy. For several weeks during this time in my pregnancy, I listened to ED. I restricted my food intake and obsessed over food. When I started my second trimester, I was ravenous. I could not stop eating. That restriction turned into constantly filling beyond fullness for most of my meals. *"I should continue restricting."* I listened to these whispers for a couple of weeks, but it was futile. I went back to that restrict-binge cycle, and I knew even as I was restricting that it was my eating disorder in my brain and not my healthy brain leading me to restrict.

Whether pregnant or not, I know that if I'm hungry, I eat. So, if there are thoughts in my brain that are guiding me towards restriction, these are eating disorder thoughts. After 2 weeks of this up and down in food intake and meeting with my therapist again, I made the active decision to stop the cycle. I decided to follow my hunger cues. My body continued to bloat and grow, but not at any different rate than it was before when I was restricting my food intake. My body needed the nourishment, and the bloating and the growing of belly faster and bigger than the previous pregnancy was completely and absolutely normal.

I was able to stay in wise mind for weeks, until a couple of people the exact same week mentioned how astonished they were that I was so big this early on in pregnancy (thinking back, 4-5 months is not that early it's half way!). One of them even joked about whether I was having twins. These were comments ED was already silently whispering in my head, so when people outside my head confirmed these thoughts, ED returned with a vengeance. I remember being at a pool gathering, being extremely anxious about wearing a bikini and eating in front of others. And I happened to be the largest woman there (all the other women were skinny). I immediately mentioned it to my husband who made an inappropriate (but much needed and welcome) joke about large things. And when I mentioned it to my best friend, she gave me a motto that I started repeating over and over in my head in order to stop ED thoughts and prevent me from relapsing again:

*"Your body is the least
interesting thing about you."*

She also reminded me about a wonderful **mirroring technique** when having thoughts of restriction. **She told me to look at my daughter and tell her that she had to stop eating because she was getting too big. Just the thought of telling my daughter that brings me to tears; the pain of even picturing me saying that to get is unbearable.** She deserves food, regardless of her size. At the same time, that mirroring technique made me so angry and frustrated with my own parents because they DID sit me down when I was eight years old and told me to stop eating because I was getting fat.

Once again, I found myself **taking action for my unborn child. The driving force behind healthy mind coming forward in my brain was to maximize my unborn child's health. I wanted to set an example for my kids starting in the womb. I**

was not going to let natural and normal body changes during a beautiful time in my life (that only happens a handful of times for most women) be ruined by my eating disorder. I was not going to spend another 4-5 months mourning the loss of my previous body.

As my body continued to grow, my family and loved ones were excited and eager that my body was changing. Lovingly, they'd continue to mention how my belly was getting bigger. As much as I was fighting my eating disorder thoughts, these comments still made ED scream in my head to take action: to stop eating even though I was hungry 24/7, and to increase the amount of physical activity I was doing. The comments made my mental battle to thrive in pregnancy a lot harder. So, **I started speaking up. I started asking people who were commenting on my body size to**

please stop. More specifically, my parents. They would mention my belly multiple times any time they visited. And they both know about my recovery, they know about the rule my first therapist gave them over 10 years ago: "no talk of food, shape, weight, or size." Yet, I still had to remind them.

Literally my dad would ask *"still?"*

"Still." I'd echo. *"It still affects me."*

"It's been so long, I thought you were over it."

"I'm over most of it, but sometimes I struggle. And these comments make my struggling worse."

I again would have to repeat this same conversation any time I saw them.

This is a technique called "broken record." You repeat yourself, almost the exact same way if needed, until people get your

message permanently. Sometimes, you repeat yourself indefinitely and that's ok. Everyone has their own issues, and they may forget what you're going through; or maybe you look like you're doing well on the outside, so they think you're doing well on the inside. Personally, after recovery I never shared relapses in thoughts or behaviors with my parents. My recovery was hard on them, and I didn't want them to worry about me, less so when I knew I'd get over my lapse in recovery eventually.

But when the comments continued and I had to use the broken-record technique again, I'd mention that I was struggling. Just that simple phrase, without any further explanation, would typically suffice for the duration of that visit. Then, next visit if I was struggling and they mentioned something, I'd use the broken-record technique again.

With each pregnancy, our bodies change at different rates and in a different way, and that's normal. This is what I used to tell my patients. As women, our bodies' set points will change with any major changes of hormones. This includes menarche, pregnancies, and menopause. It is natural and normal for our bodies to change. And even without our hormones surging at these different milestones in our lives as women, it is still normal for human bodies to change over time. There are many factors that influence our body shape and size besides genetics (access to food, developmental determinants, emotional state, prenatal care…)[4].

If you are not yet pregnant and planning to get pregnant, or if you are on earlier weeks of pregnancy, set some money aside in case you would benefit from seeing a therapist again. If you currently

have a therapist, keep seeing
him/her throughout your pregnancy.
Talk to friends, new moms, find a
local group of moms on social
media... Just like in ED recovery,
create a support network all around
you that you can fall back on in case
ED decides to come knocking again
when you least expect it.

ED and Pregnancy Brain Changes

For me, pregnancy ignited my maternal animal instincts. Even during my first pregnancy, my inner animal did everything to protect my cub at all costs. This is counterintuitive to having eating disorder thoughts increase, as a full-blow ED relapse would place my unborn child at higher risk of all sorts of complications. I started to think about why this could be. Was it just that the eating disorder voice is that strong, even after years in recovery? So, I did some research.

I already knew that eating disorders anatomically change brain structure over time[5]. For example, anorexia Nervosa can directly decrease the number of neuronal connections in the brain, resulting in a smaller brain volume. The longer the course of illness, the greater the damage, which is one of the many reasons why early intervention and recovery are so important. Makes sense. Less connections would imply less ability to think critically. So that maternal instinct would not be able to fully manifest itself if the thought cannot come to fruition given that it cannot travel through the brain into the prefrontal cortex (which plays a major role in impulse control) given there aren't enough neuronal connections[6]. In this case, the impulse to follow ED thoughts would outweigh the instinct to protect the baby in the womb because the prefrontal cortex connections (among others) are disrupted. In addition to decrease in activity on the prefrontal cortex, people with history of an eating disorder will have increased activity of the amygdala[7]. The amygdala plays a significant role in reward learning and shame processing. People with enlarged amygdalae may have increased shame about their own bodies with an inability to process reward from nourishment, for example. Translated to an eating disorder, you would have a more distorted body image while feeling rewarded when engaging in behaviors that do not support survival of the body (i.e.: restriction, purging, binging).

Regardless of how long a person has been recovered, these brain changes may be irreversible. This could lead to a particular time of stress to re-ignite old patterns in the brain that we've learned to bypass through neuroplasticity. But pregnancy also produces brain changes that could exacerbate brain changes previously there from a history of eating disorder. Particularly in pregnancy there can also be loss of neuronal connections on specific areas of the brain (the so called "mom brain" is physiologically accurate)[8]. which may compound in the previously lost connections during the eating disorder. It's speculated that the loss of brain matter during pregnancy in specific areas of the brain is to stimulate mom-to-baby attachment by decreasing mom hostility towards baby and increasing recognition of baby's social cues to best cater to his/her needs[9].

Weeks 20-27

By this point, I was tired of fighting my eating disorder thoughts. I decided to stop fighting but also not to engage in them. I spent these weeks of pregnancy completely ignoring ED thoughts in my brain and focusing on wise mind thoughts. ***"How do I want to behave to protect my baby long term?"*** was an hourly self-talk. ED would be screaming in my head every step of the way, yet I made a conscious effort to discern what my healthy mind was telling me at every instance ED would try to get my attention. I decided that fighting with ED was pointless and that the thoughts would continue to be there. It did take a lot of emotional energy to achieve this, and I found myself more easily irritable towards my loved ones. I immediately opened up to my husband and explained that I may be snappier. My goal was to protect my unborn baby.

My husband is an adult who can process that if I snap at him, it's because my plate is full (and also a bit because of something he may have done but that's beside the point). He was able to understand and support me, which made it easier to focus my energy in listening to my wise mind instead of also having to focus it on not reacting as much. Which, in turn, helped not to react towards him as much because I was able to relax knowing I was in a safe space.

If you find yourself more irritable when trying to minimize ED thoughts on your brain, it's very normal because we only have limited amount of brain power, and ED tends to destroy a lot of it (as we learned in the previous chapter). Cut yourself some grace, you're doing the best you can to protect your kids and yourself against yourself. It's normal to have these

eating disorder thoughts (and even behaviors) return during pregnancy. Whoever is part of your support circle, whether husband, best friend, parents, etc, communicate with them what you're going through internally. This will help take a huge weight off your shoulders so you can focus whatever brain power you have left in staying healthy in your recovered mind.

Sometimes it can be difficult to admit a lapse or relapse, we may feel shame. Especially if we admit it to people who have seen us recovered for a long period of time. But right now, it's more important to nourish yourself physically, emotionally, and mentally. Allow that maternal instinct to overpower the ED impulse momentarily enough to open up to your support circle, even if you haven't reached out to them in years. They are still there to support you, regardless of the time or situation.

Week 28

The time had arrived: the dreaded glucose tolerance test. To some women, it's no big deal other than the taste of the sugar drink (typically, glucola) itself, but for have of us who are recovered from an eating disorder, the glucose test has the potential of flipping our worlds upside down. If it's negative, we may feel more inclined to eat all the sugary foods for a few days, with part of our ED mind encouraging us just as if we'd learned that we lost weight when checking on the scale (to me, it gives me that same feeling even though I haven't weighed myself in over five years). If the test is positive, it means counting carbs and potentially restricting our food intake again, and we've worked really hard in our recovery to eat intuitively and accept all foods without giving them any moral values. Personally, I almost feel

ED in my brain smirking at the possibility of having to restrict my intake and triggering a relapse, and I'm terrified of that.

By 28 weeks, I had accepted my growing belly, made peace with food (again), and started embracing how powerful my body is for building a human within my uterus. Having potential of reverting back to binging on sweets for a few days or having to restrict my intake for the rest of my pregnancy was a mind-f***. I apologize for the cursing, it's the only way I can describe that feeling.

So, how do we move away from this mental struggle and prepare for the glucose tolerance test? The skill that helped me the most to avoid counting down each day and making my weeks interminable was DISTRACTION from dialectical behavioral therapy (DBT). I vested

my mind and my thoughts into mindfulness. I focused on being present in my job, in my conversations, in my life as a wife (and mom the second pregnancy). I also prepared my brain for RADICAL ACCEPTANCE (another DBT skill) in case the test was positive but tried not to even think of that possibility as it would bring about more anxiety.** But I was confident that if the test resulted positive, I had learned about radical acceptance and became quite proficient in it during my recovery to the point I knew I'd be able to use this skill regardless of my glucose test results.

**If you'd like more information about DBT, this link is useful dbtselfhelp.com. I also recommend looking up therapists in your area who have a DBT skills group to go

through each of the skills with
professional and personal support.

Weeks 29-38

As I started my third trimester during my second pregnancy, I felt great, empowered, and balanced. But within a few days, my baby bump grew quite a bit. This was likely a mix of baby having a growth spurt, having a full stomach 24/7 because I constantly felt hungry, and constipation lasting at least a week between bowel movements. People started commenting again on how big I looked, *"are you sure there's only one in there..?"* I was already starting to get insecure about my body image again and these comments had ED in my brain once again trying to convince me that since some people were saying it, it was true, so I needed to eat less and exercise more. Instead, I did **opposite of emotion action (another DBT skill)** and I continued honoring my hunger and fullness cues despite all the anxiety they caused. As I continued to eat what I wanted, I went from craving only brownies and dulce de leche, to craving a variety of foods including salads and chicken chips. Once again, my diet became more varied while intuitively eating.

My body image was still horrible, which made me feel guilty and frustrated. So many years fighting to be body neutral and now I was back to body-related negative self-talk, which typically ended with ED wanting me to believe I must therefore be worthless.

This brings me to a technique I came up with during my first year of recovery that I call "floating heads." This technique helped me become more body neutral, to the point that body shape became unimportant and insignificant. The exercise involves envisioning that everyone, including myself, has an invisibility cloak wrapped around their

shoulders so I can only see people's bodies from the neck up. This not only limits my body checks and comparison to other people's bodies, but it also has helped me to become more present and intentional during conversations with others. By focusing on the neck up, I also focus on people's eyes to help me listen intently and mindfully be in the conversation as it is happening. Before using this technique, I would focus more on the person's body than what they were telling me. I would put more emphasis on the person's body shape, weight, and size, than focusing on the depth of his/her knowledge, kindness, compassion, or whatever other trait s/he possessed that I wasn't even paying attention to.

Weeks 39-42

At this point in both of my pregnancies, my body shape became part of the background noise in my brain. Sure, I looked at my large belly with my more noticeable veins and couple of stretch marks, my mind wondering here and there how much loose skin I'd have after having each baby... But the forefront of my thoughts became awaiting the arrival of each of my children.

During my first pregnancy, I was extremely anxious as I had somehow convinced myself I was going to give birth by 38 weeks of gestational age. 38 weeks came and went, and I felt zero signs of labor. As week 40 came, I became extra anxious, as I was trying to avoid induction and during my training, most moms-to-be were induced by 39 weeks gestation. I wanted to avoid induction in order to minimize any added risk of C-section -

nothing wrong if surgical intervention is needed for delivery, but I did not feel the need to increase the risk if it was not necessary (induction increases the risk of C-section by 30%[10]). Eventually I had my baby 9 days after my due date, which I learned was very normal for a first-time mom. Typically, first pregnancy will go 7-10 past estimated date of conception if no medical interventions are initiated[11].

By 39 weeks in my second pregnancy, I was more relaxed and surrendered to the process; I knew baby would come when he and my body were ready. I was still curious and thinking about whether this time around would be similar to my prior labor and delivery experience, but I wasn't anxious about it. I wasn't concerned with my body image much either. I was thinking more about how our daughter would respond to her baby brother, particularly as she was starting to show some of the terrible two's personality traits as the delivery date got closer. I started focusing more on the family dynamics and how we'd all respond, including my husband and I as a couple: having one child had changed our relationship so much already, I wondered what having a second child would do. I wasn't anxious about it, but rather more curious and expectant.

I did have a number of instances towards the end where people would comment on my belly and body which did slightly trigger me. Random strangers commenting how I was *"all belly,"* and loved ones mentioning how *"huge"* my belly was.

Initially in the pregnancy, my ED mind would have wanted to come out and tell me to *"do something about it"* (i.e. restrict or diet) but this far along in the pregnancy (especially second pregnancy) my wise mind would automatically respond *internally*, *"of course my belly is big, I'm full term pregnant!"* The comments that had bothered me earlier on in pregnancy did not faze me now. My mind was in momma-bear-mode, ready to meet my newborn.

If you get to your later stage in pregnancy and still notice yourself focusing a lot on your body shape or size, try focusing instead in the life you've created within your womb. Picture yourself holding and loving your baby. If that's not enough to help distract you from the thoughts about your body, try envisioning how your baby will look like, how your baby will smell, visualize your baby grabbing your finger with his/her hand. Use this grounding technique to bring your brain back to wise mind and to the things you know actually matter to you in your healthy brain. Picture yourself in your new life as a mom (with one or

more kids, depending on which number pregnancy this is for you) and what you look forward to the most. You can even picture all the added stress that comes with an addition of a child to the family count. Knowing that whatever is coming, you can handle it. You've overcome so many things in your life and you've chosen recovery over and over again.

You are strong, powerful, and resilient!

References

1. Mariko Makino, Mitsuo Yasushi, and Sueharu Tsutsui "The risk of eating disorder relapse during pregnancy and after delivery and postpartum depression among women recovered from eating disorders." *BMC Pregnancy Childbirth.* 2020; 20: 323

2. T Vutyavanich, S Wongtra-ngan, R Ruangsri "Pyridoxine for nausea and vomiting of pregnancy: a randomized, double-blind, placebo-controlled trial." *Am J Obstet Gynecol.* 1995; 173(3 Pt 1):881-4.

3. Matthews A, Haas DM, O'Mathúna DP, Dowswell T "Interventions for nausea and vomiting in early pregnancy." *Cochrane Database Syst Rev.* 2015

4. *Weight Management: State of the Science and Opportunities for Military Programs* (2004) "Factors That Influence Body Weight." Institute of Medicine (US) Subcommittee on Military Weight Management.

5. Esther Walton et al "Brain Structure in Acutely Underweight and Partially Weight-Restored Individuals with Anorexia Nervosa - A Coordinated Analysis by the ENIGMA Eating Disorders Working Group." *Biological Psychiatry,* 2022; DOI: 10.1016/j.biopsych.2022.04.022.

6. Joseph E. Pizzorno and Michael T. Murray (2020) Textbook of Natural Medicine (Fifth Edition) "Prefrontal Cortex"

7. Sophie Scharner and Andreas Stengel "Alterations of brain structure and functions in anorexia nervosa" *Clinical Nutrition. 2019;* Vol. 28, P22-32.

8. Elseline Hoekzema et al "Pregnancy leads to long-lasting changes in human brain structure." *Nature Neuroscience.* 2017; vol. 20, pages 287–296.

9. Magdalena Martinez-Garcia et al "Do Pregnancy-Induced Brain Changes Reverse? The Brain of a Mother Six Years after Parturition" *Brain Sci.* 2021;11(2):168

10. Jorge Burgos et al "Induction at 41 weeks increases the risk of caesarean section in a hospital with a low rate of caesarean sections" *J Matern Fetal Neonatal Med.* 2012;25(9):1716-8

11. A R Weekes, M J Flynn "Engagement of the fetal head in primigravidae and its relationship to duration of gestation and time of onset of labour" *Br J Obstet Gynaecol.* 1975;82(1):7-11

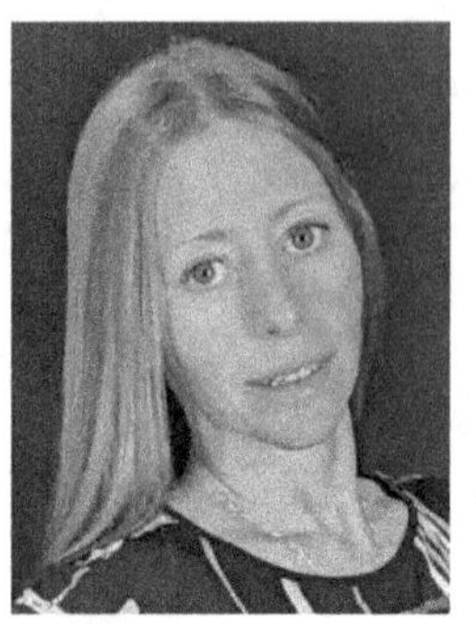

About the author: Barbara is a US-trained dual board certified family and osteopathic medicine physician, intuitive eating counselor, CrossFit level 1 trainer and adaptive athlete trainer. She lives in Central Texas with her husband, kids, and dachshund. She has been in full recovery for 5 years and started her eating disorder recovery journey over 10 years ago during medical school. Barbara is passionate about helping people succeed and thrive mind, body, and soul.

www.ingramcontent.com/pod-product-compliance
Lightning Source LLC
Chambersburg PA
CBHW061522250726

48657CB00005B/2024